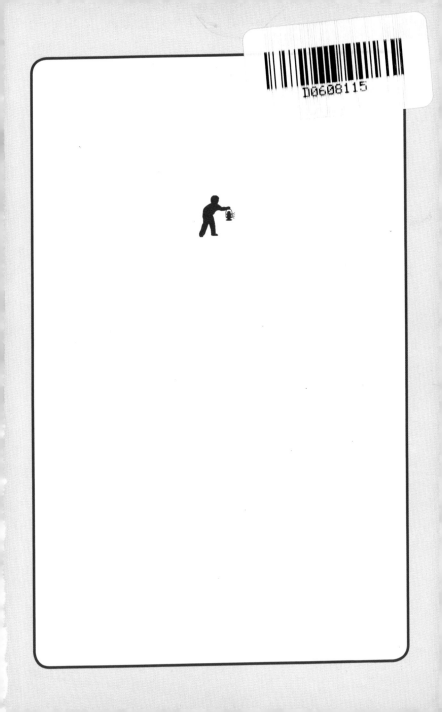

THE BOY'S FITNESS GUIDE

Frank C. Hawkins
with
Rares "Nick" Morar, A.C.E.
and
NBA Star Gheorghe Muresan

Illustrated by J.C. Hawkins

theboysguide.com

Boy's Guide Books, LLC
An imprint of Big Book Press

The boy's fitness guide: a physical fitness and health book
for young men / by Frank C. Hawkins, Rares Morar, and
Gheorghe Muresan. Illustrated by J.C. Hawkins—1st ed.
1. Boys—Physical fitness and health—Juvenile literature.
2. Boys and exercise—Juvenile literature.

Printed in Hong Kong

Library of Congress Control Number: 2007910141
ISBN-13: 978-0-9793219-1-7
ISBN-10: 0-9793219-1-3

"Commit to be fit."

—Anonymous

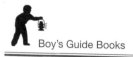

Dear Friend,

There is no more important decision you will make as a young man than to pursue the goal of being physically fit. Your commitment to exercise, good nutrition, and caring for your body will give you a lifetime of health and vitality.

Decide now to make physical fitness a life-long habit. Fitness has given me the opportunity to play professional basketball—to excel in life. And being physically fit has rewarded me with confidence and self-esteem. It will do the same for you.

This book lays out the roadmap to physical fitness. Each of the three essential stops along the way—exercise, nutrition, and body care—is covered in detail. You need ambition and determination to make it work—in a word, guts. I know you can do it.

Sincerely, #77

Gheorghe Muresan

CONTENTS

CIRCLE
OF FITNESS

Physical fitness is a way of life—a commitment to exercise, eat right, and care for your body.

Being fit has many rewards. Your body is healthy and strong. Your weight is proportional to your height. You feel good about yourself. You're alert, able to think clearly. And you look your best.

Promise yourself to make an effort each and every day to be physically fit. It's fun, and the results will surprise you.

Let's get started! There's no better time to begin than right now.

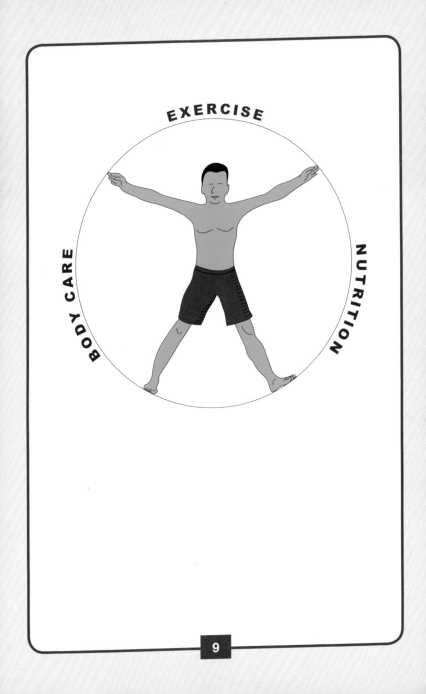

MUSCLES MAKE IT HAPPEN

You have more than 600 muscles in your body. Some muscles are called involuntary muscles because you can't control what they do. Involuntary muscles make your heart, stomach, and intestines work. They do their jobs without you even thinking about them.

You also have muscles you can control, such as those in your arms, legs, and back. They are called voluntary muscles. Working together with your skeleton, voluntary muscles give you the ability to shoot a basketball, kick a soccer ball, and shadow box.

Voluntary muscles are divided into 14 major groups. Let's take a look at them.

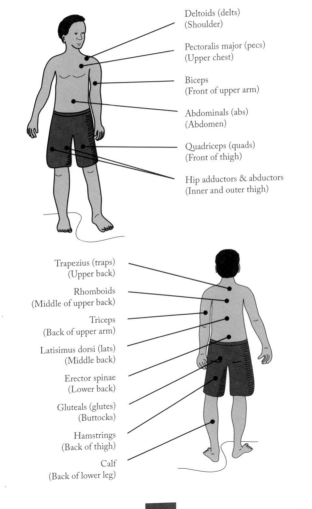

Deltoids (delts)
(Shoulder)

Pectoralis major (pecs)
(Upper chest)

Biceps
(Front of upper arm)

Abdominals (abs)
(Abdomen)

Quadriceps (quads)
(Front of thigh)

Hip adductors & abductors
(Inner and outer thigh)

Trapezius (traps)
(Upper back)

Rhomboids
(Middle of upper back)

Triceps
(Back of upper arm)

Latisimus dorsi (lats)
(Middle back)

Erector spinae
(Lower back)

Gluteals (glutes)
(Buttocks)

Hamstrings
(Back of thigh)

Calf
(Back of lower leg)

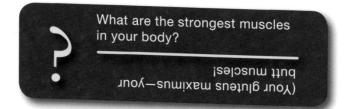

Moving your muscles takes lots of energy. Just like a car burns gasoline to make it go, your body burns sugar and fat to make you go. Here's how it works:

- Nutrients from the food you eat are absorbed through your intestines.

- The nutrients make their way to your liver where they are converted to a simple sugar (also called glucose).

- The glucose is released into your blood where it moves through your circulatory system to the places it's needed, such as your muscles, organs, and tissues.

- Any glucose (now in the form of glycogen) that isn't used up is stored in your muscles and liver.

- If you have more glycogen than your body can store, your body converts the extra into body fat.

EXERCISE— THE BIG PICTURE

Developing your body's flexibility, endurance, and strength through regular exercise is an essential part of being physically fit. If you want to stand out in a sport, or you just want to look and feel your best, exercise will make it happen.

EXERCISE DEVELOPS FLEXIBILITY, ENDURANCE, AND STRENGTH.

It's important to develop your body to its full potential. Many young men are mainly interested in building up their muscles. But building only muscular strength and ignoring flexibility and endurance is not the path to physical fitness.

Just playing basketball, for example, won't make you physically fit. To play basketball well, you need to develop your flexibility, endurance, and strength. That's why coaches insist on stretching, as well as aerobic and resistance exercises.

HOW IT ALL FITS TOGETHER		
YOUR GOAL	HOW TO GET IT	WHAT HAPPENS
Perform your best and avoid injury and muscle cramps.	Stretching	Improves muscle and joint *flexibility.*
Play soccer without getting out of breath.	Aerobic exercise	Builds up *endurance* by increasing heart and lung capacity.
Tone your body and strengthen your muscles.	Resistance exercise	Increases muscular *strength* and conditioning.

Tips...Tips...

Here are some tips on how to start exercising and how to keep your exercise program going:

- Decide on your exercise goals. What do you want to achieve? For example, if you want to improve your endurance, emphasize aerobic exercises. If you want to tone your body, emphasize resistance exercises. Make your goals reasonable and realistic.

- Develop an exercise plan based on your goals. Be sure your plan includes warm-up and stretching (flexibility), aerobic (endurance), and resistance (strength) exercises. To excel in any one requires work in all three.

- Set up a regular exercise schedule and stick to it. You are more likely to continue exercising when you have a schedule to follow.

- Begin slowly and progress little by little. If you're just starting a program, start with easy exercises. Gradually work up to more advanced exercises.

- Keep track of your progress by writing it down.

- Get a friend to exercise with you.

- Consider working with a coach or trainer to motivate you and provide instruction.

- Try to exercise three to four days a week for about 30 to 45 minutes each time. It's important to allow your body time to recover between workouts. Don't overdo it.

WARMING UP AND STRETCHING

No matter whether you're shooting some hoops with friends or competing in a championship soccer match, the first two things you should do are warm up and stretch. Together, warming up and stretching help you perform your best without pain or injury.

FLEXIBILITY HELPS YOU JUMP HIGHER, REACH FURTHER, AND RUN FASTER.

Jogging, shadow boxing, and jumping jacks are great ways to warm up. They'll get your heart beating faster and increase blood flow to your muscles and joints. Sweating and breathing faster than normal are signs you're warmed up.

Stretching after you're warmed up makes your muscles and joints more flexible, preventing injuries and stopping your muscles from cramping. Flexibility also allows you to move your muscles through their full range of motion. That helps you jump higher, reach further, and run faster.

Tips...Tips...

Some good warm-up and stretching tips to know are:

- Warm up before you stretch.
- Move your joints to get your body's natural lubrication (synovial fluid) going. Rotate your wrists and

ankles, bend your elbows and knees, and roll your shoulders. Make sure the movements are slow and controlled and that your joints move through their full range of motion.

- Stretch all your major muscle groups, beginning with your upper body, then your middle body, and finally your lower body.

- Do each stretch at least once.

- Breathe normally—in through your nose and out through your mouth. Don't hold your breath.

- Maintain the correct form and body posture.

- Gently put tension on your muscles.

- Stretching should feel good and not cause pain. If it does, stop.

- Take about 15 minutes to warm up and stretch.

STRETCHES

To improve flexibility, prevent injury, and increase performance.

Upper Back Stretch (Upper Body)

1. Intertwine your fingers with your palms turned away from you.

2. Reach out, rolling your shoulders forward and extending your arms as far as possible.

3. Hold the stretch 10 to 15 seconds.

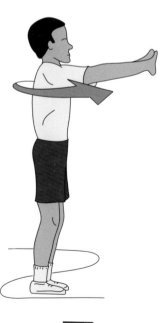

Chest Stretch (Upper Body)

1. Clasp your hands behind your back.

2. Keep your elbows straight.

3. Rotate your shoulders backward, squeezing your shoulder blades together.

4. Hold the stretch 10 to 15 seconds.

(For a greater challenge, look up while doing the stretch.)

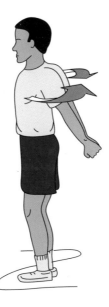

Biceps Stretch (Upper Body)

1. Lift your arms to shoulder height at your sides.

2. Rotate your wrists so your palms face behind you.

3. Hold the stretch 10 to 15 seconds.

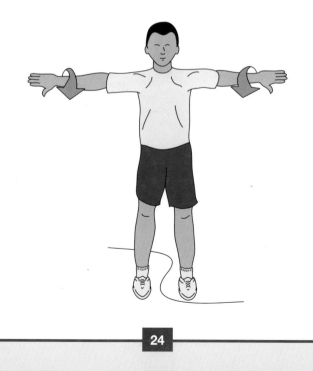

Triceps Stretch (Upper Body)

1. Start with your arms overhead.

2. Grab your left elbow with your right hand.

3. Slowly pull your elbow toward the back of your head.

4. Hold the stretch 10 to 15 seconds.

5. Repeat on the other side.

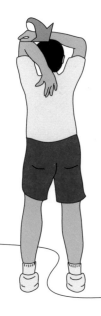

Shoulder Stretch (Upper Body)

1. Cross your right arm over your chest.

2. With your left hand, gently pull your right elbow toward your left shoulder. Keep your right arm straight.

3. Hold the stretch 10 to 15 seconds.

4. Repeat on the other side.

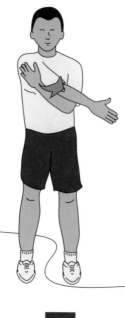

Neck Stretch (Upper Body)

1. Begin with your head in its normal upright position.

2. Gently tilt your head sideways, first to the right, then left, front, and back.

3. Hold the stretch in each direction 10 to 15 seconds.

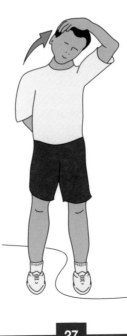

Side Stretch (Middle Body)

1. Stand with your feet shoulder-width apart.

2. Place your right hand behind your back and your left arm overhead.

3. Reach up with your left hand and lean to the right.

4. Hold the stretch 10 to 15 seconds.

5. Repeat on the other side.

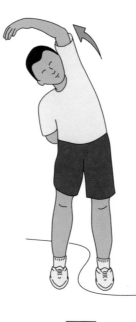

Back Stretch (Middle Body)

1. Stand with your feet shoulder width apart and your knees slightly bent.

2. Put your hands on your thighs.

3. Gently arch your back, rolling your shoulders and leaning forward slightly.

4. Hold the stretch 10 to 15 seconds.

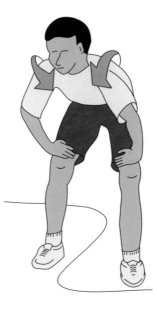

Quadriceps Stretch (Lower Body)

1. Keeping your back straight, grab the top of your left foot with your left hand.

2. Pull your heel toward your butt.

3. Hold the stretch 10 to 15 seconds.

4. Repeat on the other side.

(For a greater challenge, balance on one foot without holding on to anything for support.)

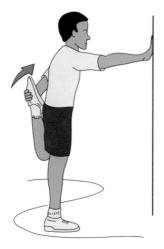

Calf Stretch (Lower Body)

1. Lean against a wall with your hands.

2. Bend your right knee.

3. Move your left foot back, keeping your leg straight, while pressing your heel toward the floor.

4. Move your hips forward until you feel tension in your left calf muscle.

5. Hold the stretch 10 to 15 seconds.

6. Repeat on the other side.

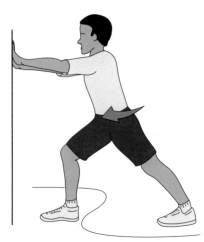

Hamstrings Stretch (Lower Body)

1. Sit on the floor with your feet together and legs straight.

2. Grab your ankles and lean forward, trying to touch your forehead to the tops of your legs.

3. Hold the stretch 10 to 15 seconds.

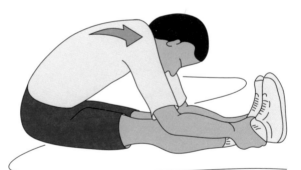

Inner Thigh Stretch (Lower Body)

1. Sit with the soles of your feet flat against each other.

2. Hold your ankles, with your elbows gently pressing your knees toward the floor.

3. Lean forward, lowering your chest toward your feet until you feel your inner thighs stretch.

4. Hold the stretch 10 to 15 seconds.

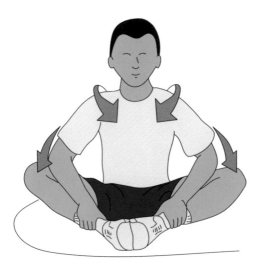

Outer Thigh Stretch (Lower Body)

1. Sit on the floor with your left leg straight out in front of you.

2. Cross your right foot over and place it on the outside of your left knee.

3. With your right hand on the floor behind you, bring your left elbow across your body and place it on the outside of your right thigh.

4. Twist your body as you look over your right shoulder.

5. Hold the stretch 10 to 15 seconds.

6. Repeat on the other side.

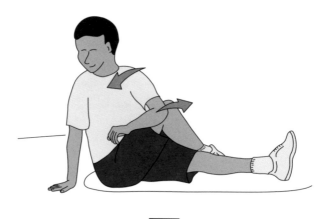

AEROBIC EXERCISE

Imagine you're playing soccer. It's the second period and you've been running hard for the last 15 minutes. You're working up a good sweat, you're breathing hard, and your heart is pounding. That's aerobic exercise.

AEROBIC FITNESS MEANS YOU CAN PLAY SPORTS LONGER WITHOUT GETTING TIRED OR OUT OF BREATH.

When you breathe, your lungs take oxygen from the air and put it into your blood. Your heart pumps this oxygen-rich blood through your blood vessels to your muscles. Your muscles use the oxygen to burn sugar (in the form of glycogen) and fat to give you energy. To keep you running for the whole soccer game, your muscles demand more and more oxygen-rich blood. That makes your heart beat faster and faster to keep up.

Aerobic exercise involves continual rhythmic movement of your large muscles, especially your leg and buttocks muscles. Aerobic exercise is lower intensity exercise that you do for longer periods of time. For example, running a long distance at an average pace is an aerobic activity. But sprinting a short distance is not because of its high intensity (See *Resistance Exercise*). And swimming is an aerobic activity. But golf and baseball, with their more frequent breaks, are not.

With regular aerobic exercise, your heart muscle and the muscles that move air in and out of your lungs will grow stronger. As that happens, they'll meet your voluntary muscles' demands for oxygen without as much effort. And, over time, all your muscles will begin to use oxygen more efficiently. That means you'll burn more sugar and fat, be more aerobically fit, and play soccer—or any sport you choose—longer without getting tired or out of breath.

There are many kinds of aerobic exercise. Some, like riding a stationary bike, are done only for the aerobic benefit. Others, like basketball, are played for fun and competition and the aerobic benefit is a welcome result.

One last thing: After hard aerobic exercise, it's a good idea to walk around for a few minutes to get your breathing back to normal and slow your heartbeat down. If time allows, it's also a good idea to stretch your major muscle groups again. Stretching after you exercise will stop your muscles from cramping and getting sore.

Tips...Tips...

Here are some good aerobic activities:

- Bicycling.
- Basketball.
- Cross-country skiing.
- Hiking.
- In-line, ice, and roller skating.
- Running and jogging.
- Jumping rope.
- Ice hockey.
- Soccer.
- Rugby.
- Lacrosse.
- Swimming.
- Stair climbing.

Your Heart Rate

You already know that your heart beats faster when you're exercising and slower when you're resting. But just how much faster and how much slower does it beat?

The main objectives of aerobic exercise are to get you breathing faster and speed up your heart rate. But to get the most benefit from the aerobic exercise, you must keep your heart beating within a certain range—not too high and not too low.

To make sure that happens, you need to know three numbers:

1. Resting Heart Rate (RHR)

2. Maximum Heart Rate (MHR)

3. Target Heart Rate (THR)

FIRST, let's determine your RHR by counting how many times your heart beats in one minute. You can feel your heart beat, or pulse, anywhere there's an artery near the surface of your skin. The two best places are on either side of your neck just below your jaw line (carotid artery) and the inside of either wrist on the thumb side (radial artery).

Here's how to measure your RHR:

STEP 1.
Relax. The best time to measure your RHR is in the morning before you get out of bed.

STEP 2.
Lightly press your index and middle fingers on the arteries in either your neck or wrist. (Don't

use your thumb to measure your pulse rate because the artery in your thumb pulses so strongly that you may count its pulse by accident.)

Step 3.

Count the number of pulses you feel in 10 seconds. Begin your count 0 – 1 – 2 – 3 – 4 – and so on.

Step 4.

Multiply by 6 the number of pulses you counted in 10 seconds. (For example, 12 pulses x 6 = RHR of 72 beats per minute, or bpm.)

As your aerobic fitness increases, your RHR will go down. This lets you measure your beginning aerobic fitness level and chart your progress over time.

Compare your RHR to the numbers in the following table. Where do you fit in?

Age	Resting Heart Rate (beats per minute)
Newborn	120 to 160
0 to 5 months	90 to 140
6 to 12 months	80 to 140
1 to 3 years	80 to 130
4 to 5 years	80 to 120
6 to 10 years	70 to 110
11 to 14 years	60 to 105
Over 14 years	60 to 100

Second, calculate your maximum heart rate, or MHR, using this formula:

220 − YOUR AGE = MHR

Example: If you are 14 years old, your MHR would be 206 beats per minute (220 − 14 = 206 bpm).

Third, now that you know your RHR and MHR, you can calculate your target heart rate, or THR. There is an upper "intensity" and a lower "intensity" THR. Between them is *the zone* in which your heart and

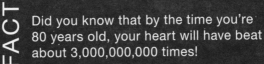

lungs get the most benefit from aerobic exercise. Your THR zone is generally between 60% and 85% of your MHR.

Use the following formula (The Karvonen method) to calculate your upper and lower THR:

((MHR – RHR) x % Intensity) + RHR = THR

Example: If your MHR is 206 bpm and your RHR is 72 bpm, you would calculate your upper and lower THR as follows:

<u>**Lower intensity (60%):**</u>
((206 – 72) x 0.60) + 72 = 152 bpm

<u>**Upper intensity (85%):**</u>
((206 – 72) x 0.85) + 72 = 186 bpm

This means your THR zone is 152 bpm to 186 bpm. Take your pulse periodically as you exercise and adjust the intensity of your exercise to stay within the 60% to 85% range.

When you first start doing aerobic exercise, aim for the lowest part of your THR zone (60%). Slowly build up to the higher part of your THR zone. After six or more months of regular exercise, you may be able to exercise comfortably at the 85% upper intensity. However, remember that you don't have to exercise that hard to stay in shape.

RESISTANCE EXERCISE

Let's do an experiment with your arm muscles. First, stand with your arms at your side. Bend your right arm at the elbow, touching your fingers to your shoulder and then returning your arm to its starting position. Repeat the movement 10 times. Your arm isn't tired, is it? The reason is that your arm muscles didn't have to work very hard to lift your arm up and down.

Now, repeat the exercise holding a bottle of water in your right hand. This time your arm muscles feel tired. The reason is *resistance*. To lift the water bottle, your arm muscles had to overcome (resist) the weight of the water bottle. The heavier the bottle, the more resistance, and the harder your muscles have to work. Resistance exercise is *anaerobic*, meaning it is "without oxygen." Anaerobic exercise, like weight lifting and sprinting, uses muscles at *high* intensity for *short* periods of time (2 to 3 minutes), as opposed to *aerobic* exercise, which is *low* intensity for *long* periods of time (15 or more minutes).

The energy for anaerobic exercise comes from glycogen stored in your muscles.

FACT

Timing is everything. Before you reach puberty, resistance exercise will tone your body but it won't make your muscles bigger. That's because your body doesn't start making the hormones you need to build muscles until puberty. In the meantime, eat healthy foods and stay active. That will keep you strong and ready to start building muscles when your body is ready.

Working Your Muscles

Now, let's take another look at your voluntary muscles: the ones you use to do resistance exercises. Different exercises work different muscle groups.

MAJOR MUSCLE GROUP	LOCATION	EXERCISE
Deltoids (delts) a. Anterior delts	a. Front of shoulder.	a. Push-up, bench press, front dumbbell raise.
b. Medial delts	b. Middle of shoulder.	b. Side dumbbell raise.
c. Posterior delts	c. Back of shoulder.	c. Rear dumbbell raise.
Pectoralis major (pecs)	Upper chest.	Push-up, chin-up, regular and incline bench press.
Trapezius (traps)	Upper back.	Upright row, shoulder shrug, pull-up.
Rhomboids	Middle of upper back.	Chin-up, bent-over dumbbell row.

Major Muscle Group	Location	Exercise
Latisimus dorsi (lats)	Middle back.	Pull-up, chin-up, dip, bent-over dumbbell row.
Erector spinae	Lower back.	Back extension.
Biceps	Front of upper arm.	Curls with barbell or dumbbell, chin-up.
Triceps	Back of upper arm.	Push-up, dip, triceps extension, overhead press, bench press.
Abdominals (abs)	Abdomen.	Crunch, leg lift, plank.
Gluteals (glutes)	Buttocks.	Squat, lunge, step-up.
Quadriceps (quads)	Front of thigh.	Squat, lunge, step-up.
Hamstrings	Back of thigh.	Squat, lunge.
Hip adductors and abductors	Inner and outer thigh.	Side-lying leg lift.
Calves	Back of lower leg.	Calf raise.

As you make your list of resistance exercises you're going to do, here are some important things to consider:

Selection and Sequence

Include at least one exercise from each major muscle group on your list. Start your exercise session with compound exercises that involve two or more joint movements and work several muscle groups at once, like bench presses and squats. Work toward isolation exercises that primarily involve just one joint movement and one muscle group, like biceps curls and leg extensions. This approach allows you to do the most demanding exercises when your muscles are the least tired. For example, you'll use better form on your bench presses if you do them before exhausting your triceps doing triceps extensions.

Sets and Reps

A "set" is a group of exercise movements done one after another without resting. The number of times you do the movement is called a "rep" (repetition). If your plan is to do 3 sets of 12 biceps curls, begin by curling the weight 12 times in a row. That finishes the first set of 12 reps. Put the weights down and rest about a minute or so. Do the same for the second and third sets, and then you're done!

Speed

A good pace for doing one repetition is 1 to 3 seconds for the lifting part of the exercise and 3 to 4 seconds for the lowering part. If you lift and lower the weight too fast, it's the momentum of the weight, not your muscle, that's doing most of the work. That won't build up your muscles as fast as doing the exercise the right way. And don't jerk the weight to get it moving. It puts a lot of unnecessary stress on your muscles and joints and can injure you.

Resistance

The number of repetitions you do for each exercise will depend on how much resistance (weight) you're using. Maximum resistance is the most weight you can lift once using the proper form. Don't do resistance exercises with the most weight you can lift. Get your coach or trainer to help you determine the right weight for you. It will be different for every exercise. A good rule of thumb is to do 3 sets of 8 to 12 repetitions using 65% to 85% of your maximum resistance. Training with more than 85% of your maximum resistance can injure you. Training with less than 65% of your maximum resistance won't tone your body or strengthen your muscles very much.

Progression

As you do more and more resistance exercises, your muscles will develop and get used to the exercises. To continue toning your body and strengthening your muscles, you'll need to slowly increase the resistance and the repetitions. Start out with a weight that allows you to do at least 8 repetitions. Once you can do 12 repetitions with that weight, increase the weight to the next level. Now, you're doing 8 repetitions with the heavier weight. Just like before, work up to 12 repetitions with the heavier weight, then increase the weight and go back to doing 8 repetitions. The idea is to slowly increase repetitions and resistance, so you'll continue to tone your body and strengthen your muscles.

Frequency

When you do resistance exercises, your muscle tissue "breaks down" under the strain of the exercise and grows back bigger and stronger. The process is known as hypertrophy. Your muscles recover and get stronger during the rest period between workouts, not while you're exercising. You can exercise every day, just don't work the same muscle groups two days in a row.

RESISTANCE EXERCISES

The secret to toning your body and building muscular strength.

Bench Press with Dumbbells (Compound Exercise)

1. Begin with your arms out to your side and bent 90 degrees. Your palms should be facing your feet and your wrists straight.

2. Push the weights up until your elbows are almost straight. Don't lock your elbows or bow your back.

3. Slowly return to the starting position.

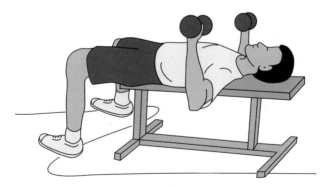

Dip (Compound Exercise)

1. Place your hands on the dip bars with your arms straight. Your feet should not touch the floor.

2. Lower your body by bending your elbows until your arms are bent at a 90 degree angle.

3. Keep your elbows next to your body.

4. Slowly return to the starting position.

(If you don't have dip bars, support yourself between two chairs with your heels resting on the floor in front of you.)

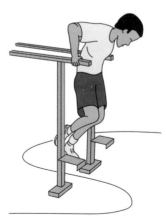

Chin-Up* (Compound Exercise)

1. Grip the bar with your hands shoulder-width apart using an underhand hold (palms facing inward). Your feet should not touch the floor.

2. Raise your body until your chin clears the bar.

3. Slowly return to the starting position.

Pull-ups are the same except with an overhand hold.

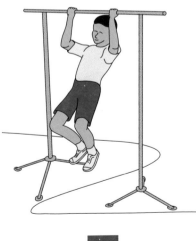

Push-Up (Compound Exercise)

1. Lie face down on the floor with your hands under your shoulders and your legs straight.

2. Straighten your arms and raise yourself to the starting position. Keep your back and legs straight.

3. Lower yourself until your body is parallel to the floor. Don't touch the floor.

(Support your body weight on your knees to make the exercise less challenging. For more of a challenge, elevate your feet.)

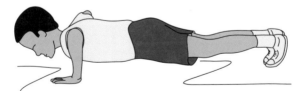

Bent-Over Dumbbell Row
(Compound Exercise)

1. Hold the weight in your right hand with your arm hanging straight down. Keep your back straight and parallel to the weight bench by looking up.

2. Keeping your elbow in, pull the weight up until your upper arm is aligned with your back and parallel to the weight bench.

3. Slowly return to the starting position.

4. Switch sides after each set.

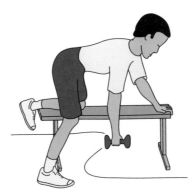

Back Extension (Compound Exercise)

1. Lie face down with your legs together and straight, and your arms stretched out in front, palms on the floor.

2. Raise your head and shoulders off the mat as high as possible. Do not tense your shoulder muscles.

3. Slowly return to the starting position.

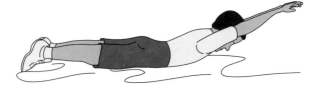

Lunge (Compound Exercise)

1. Stand with your feet about 12 inches apart.

2. Step about 2 to 3 feet forward with your right leg.

3. Lower your body until your left knee is 3 to 4 inches from the floor and your right knee is over your ankle. Keep your back straight.

4. Slowly return to the starting position.

5. Repeat, leading with your left leg this time.

(Hold dumbbells at your side for a greater challenge.)

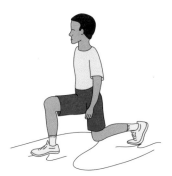

Squat (Compound Exercise)

1. Stand with your feet slightly greater than shoulder-width apart.

2. Lower your body, bending through the hips, knees, and ankles until your knees are bent 90 degrees. Keep your back straight.

3. Return to the starting position.

(Hold dumbbells at your side for a greater challenge.)

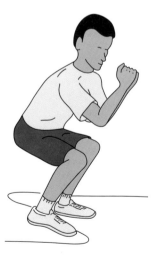

Step-Up* (Compound Exercise)

1. Step up with your right leg. Then step up with your left leg.

2. Step down with your right leg, then your left leg.

3. Repeat, starting with your left leg this time.

(Hold light weights for more of a challenge.)

*Knee-high steps work more of your quadriceps. Higher steps work more of your gluteals.

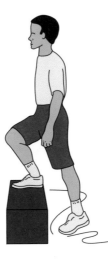

Plank (Compound Exercise)

1. Lie face down resting on your forearms, hands clasped.

2. Push off the floor, raising up onto your toes and resting on your elbows.

3. Keep your back straight. Don't hold your breath.

4. Hold the position as long as you can.

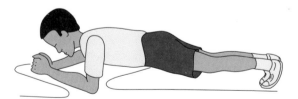

Biceps Curl (Isolation Exercise)

1. Begin with the weights at your sides, palms facing in, and arms straight.

2. Curl the weight up by bending your elbow, rotating your forearm until it is vertical and your palm faces your shoulder.

3. Slowly return to the starting position.

4. Alternate sides* to finish the set.

Another option is to lift the weights at the same time. Be sure to keep your back straight when using this technique.

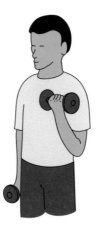

Triceps Extension (Isolation Exercise)

1. Lie on your back with your feet flat on the floor or bench.

2. Raise your right arm toward the ceiling, supporting your arm just below the elbow with your left hand.

3. Bend your right elbow, bringing the weight toward your shoulder.

4. Slowly return to the starting position.

5. Switch sides after each set.

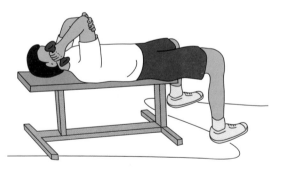

Front Dumbbell Raise
(Isolation Exercise)

1. Stand with your arms hanging in front of you, palms facing your body.

2. Keeping your elbow straight, raise your right arm in front of you until it reaches just above shoulder level.

3. Lower your right arm while raising your left arm. Keep your back straight.

4. Slowly return to the starting position after the set.

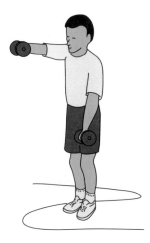

Shoulder Shrug (Isolation Exercise)

1. Stand with your arms by your side, palms facing your body.

2. Lift your shoulders up toward the back of your head.

3. Keep your arms straight, knees slightly bent, and chest up.

4. Slowly return to the starting position.

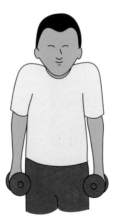

Crunch (Isolation Exercise)

1. Lie on your back with your legs bent.

2. Clasp your hands behind your head.

3. Lift your chest toward your knees until your shoulders come off the floor.

4. Slowly return to the starting position.

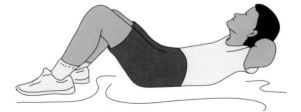

Leg Lift (Isolation Exercise)

1. Lie on your back with your arms by your side, palms down.

2. Bring your right leg up as high as possible.

3. Keep your leg straight and your back flat on the floor.

4. Slowly return to the starting position.

5. Alternate sides to finish the set.

(Bend your knees to make the exercise less difficult.)

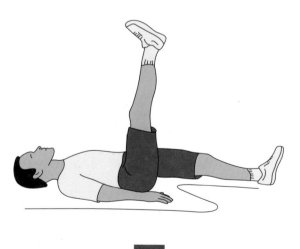

Leg Extension (Isolation Exercise)

1. Sit on a chair or weight bench high enough so your feet don't touch the floor.

2. Raise your legs until they're almost fully extended.

3. Slowly return to the starting position.

(Use ankle weights for a greater challenge.)

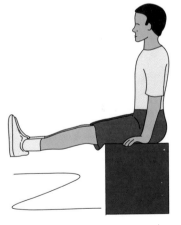

Side-Lying Leg Lift (Isolation Exercise)

1. Lie on your side with your legs one on top of the other.

2. Raise your top leg as high as you can. Keep your leg straight and your hips stacked.

3. Slowly return to the starting position.

4. Switch sides after each set.

(Use ankle weights for a greater challenge.)

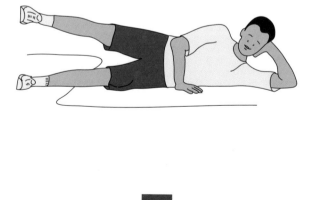

Calf Raise (Isolation Exercise)

1. Stand with your feet slightly apart.

2. Rise up onto your toes. Keep your back straight.

3. Slowly return to the starting position.

(Hold dumbbells at your sides for a greater challenge. Or stand on a step and let your heels drop below the level of your toes for a greater range of motion.)

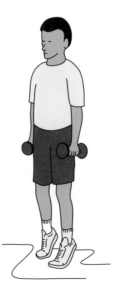

NUTRITION

Food is fuel for your body just as gasoline is fuel for a car. How quickly a car uses gasoline depends on how far and how fast it's driven. In just the same way, how quickly you use food energy depends on what physical activities you do and how long you do them.

> **FACT**
>
> Calories give your body energy. But if you eat more calories than your body needs, the leftover calories are converted to fat. And too much fat leads to health problems, such as diabetes and high blood pressure.

Food energy is measured in calories. When you hear that a food or drink contains 100 calories, it's a way of telling you how much energy it will give you. A cup of shredded lettuce, for example, has less than 10 calories. A cup of peanuts has over 850 calories.

How many calories you need depends on your age, body size, and how physically active you are. The best way to make sure you are not getting too many or too few calories is to check your weight from time to time. If you're staying within your ideal weight range (see *Body Mass Index*), you're probably consuming the right amount of calories.

The table on the next page has guidelines on the average number of calories your body needs each day. Remember that these numbers are averages.

Age	Average Calorie Intake/Day
7 – 10 years	2,000
11 – 14 years	2,500
15 – 18 years	3,000

Body Weight

Not everyone grows and develops on the same schedule. During puberty, your body makes hormones that set off physical changes, such as muscle growth, height spurts, and weight gain. The changes will continue for several years once they start. On average, you can expect to grow as much as 10 inches during puberty before reaching your full adult height.

Most young men gain weight quickly during puberty as the amounts of muscle, fat, and bone in their bodies increase. All that new weight gain is fine—as long as your body fat, muscle, and bones are in the right proportion. Remember, too, that some young men start developing as early as age 8 and others not until age 14 or later. For that reason, two young men who are the same height and age may have very different weights.

> **FACT**
>
> Every extra pound of body fat requires that your heart pump blood through another quarter mile of blood vessels.

Body Mass Index

Body Mass Index, or BMI, is the best way to figure out if your height and weight are in the right proportion. BMI is a formula that doctors use to calculate body fat based on your weight and height. After calculating your BMI, it's plotted on a chart that tells you whether you're underweight, average weight, or overweight.

Figuring out your BMI is kind of complicated, especially if you're in your teens (because of puberty). If your weight is of interest or concern to either you or your parents, ask your doctor to help you calculate your BMI. Your doctor is able to do more than assess just your current weight. He or she can also look at your BMI over time and determine whether you are at risk of becoming overweight. Knowing the risks early allows you to make changes in your diet and exercise before body weight becomes a problem.

Also remember that while BMI is a good indicator of body fat, it doesn't always tell the whole story. Someone can have a high BMI because he has a large frame or a lot of muscle (like a bodybuilder or athlete) instead of excess fat. Likewise, a small person with a small frame may have a normal BMI but could still have too much body fat. These are other good reasons to talk with your doctor about your BMI.

Eating and Drinking

Before You Exercise

Before you exercise, it's a good idea to consume foods that are high in carbohydrates, such as bananas, bagels, or fruit juice. Your body breaks these foods down quickly to provide glucose to your muscles. Researchers have found that eating high-carbohydrate foods 1 to 4 hours before exercising provides plenty of blood glucose for your working muscles. And don't forget to drink plenty of water before exercising to keep your body properly hydrated.

While You Exercise

Perspiration (sweat) drains your body of fluids. The harder you exercise and the warmer it is, the more you sweat. And the more you sweat, the more important it is to replace the fluids you've lost. Drink plenty of fluids as you exercise—at least half a cup for every 20 minutes of exercise.

After You Exercise

Drink plenty of fluids and eat a nutritious, balanced meal with lots of carbohydrate-rich foods, such as grains, pastas, potatoes, vegetables, and fruits.

Fluids Before, During, and After

Water is the most important nutrient—your life-blood. You can survive a month without food, but only 3 to 7 days without water. Drink water before, during, and after exercising. Your body needs it. If you exercise hard and non-stop for more than 90 minutes, you should replace the electrolytes and carbohydrates you lost through your sweat. There are special "sports" drinks that will do the job, or you can make a homemade sports drink by mixing 2 to 4 teaspoons of sugar, 1/4 teaspoon of salt, and some flavoring (like a teaspoon of lemon juice) in 8 ounces of water.

Snacks

Snacks are a great way to refuel. Choose snacks from different food groups—a glass of low-fat milk and a few graham crackers, an apple or celery sticks with peanut butter and raisins, or some dry cereal. Cookies, chips, and candy are OK every once in a while, but only if you balance your food choices. Don't eat too much of any one food. You don't have to give up hamburgers, french fries, and ice cream; just be smart about how often and how much of them you eat.

Vitamins and Minerals

Here are the main vitamins and minerals your body needs and the foods you can eat to get them.

VITAMINS AND MINERALS	WHAT IT DOES	WHERE TO GET IT
Vitamin A	Prevents and fights infections. Helps you see. Helps your bones grow.	Carrots, pumpkin, sweet potatoes, cantaloupe, red grapefruit, apricots, broccoli, and spinach.
B Vitamins	Gives you energy, muscle tone, and healthy hair, skin, and eyes.	Meat, fish, chicken, whole-wheat bread, green vegetables, dried beans, peas, and soybeans.
Vitamin C	Fights infection and heals cuts. Helps you have healthy skin, bones, teeth, and blood vessels.	Oranges (or orange juice), strawberries, tomatoes, broccoli, green vegetables, potatoes, and cantaloupe.
Vitamin D	Forms and maintains strong bones.	Cheese, eggs, fish, and fortified cereals.

Vitamins and Minerals	What It Does	Where to Get It
Vitamin E	Keeps your skin, heart, nerves, muscles, and red blood cells healthy.	Wheat germ, corn, nuts, seeds, olives, spinach, asparagus, and leafy vegetables.
Vitamin K	Maintains healthy bones and teeth. Stops cuts from bleeding.	Cabbage, cauliflower, spinach, soybeans, and cereals.
Calcium	Builds strong bones and teeth.	Cheese, milk, yogurt, leafy green vegetables, and calcium-fortified foods, such as orange juice and cereals.
Iron	Builds red blood cells and moves oxygen from your lungs to the rest of your body.	Red meat, potatoes, eggs, beans, raisins, and whole-grain bread.

VITAMINS AND MINERALS	WHAT IT DOES	WHERE TO GET IT
Potassium	Keeps your muscles and nervous system in good shape.	Bananas, broccoli, tomatoes, oranges, beans, peas, and peanuts.
Zinc	Fights illness and infection.	Beef, pork, beans, peas, and peanuts.

FACT

Some young men supplement their diet with vitamin and mineral pills. The pills are intended to boost your health. But if you take too many pills too often they are anything but healthy. So be careful to follow the directions on the label. Just remember that vitamin and mineral pills are not a substitute for a proper diet.

GO, SLOW, WHOA

The U.S. National Heart, Lung, and Blood Institute has a chart about GO, SLOW, and WHOA foods and drinks.

GO foods and drinks are the lowest in fat, sugar, and calories. They are rich in vitamins, minerals, and other nutrients important to your health. They help you grow strong and healthy.

SLOW foods and drinks are higher in fat, added sugar, and calories than GO foods. They're not as good for you.

WHOA foods and drinks are the highest in fat, added sugar, and calories. They'll hurt your health and fitness if you eat them too often.

Protein Supplements

True or False: Eating lots of extra protein-rich foods, taking protein supplements, and exercising as hard as you can will tone your body and build muscular strength. FALSE!

It's true that your body needs protein to grow and develop properly. But a nutritious, balanced diet that includes

Go, Slow, and Whoa Foods and Drinks

GO: Eat anytime.

SLOW: Eat sometimes, at most several times a week.

WHOA: Eat only once in a while or for special treats.

	GO	SLOW	WHOA
Vegetables	Almost all fresh, frozen, and canned vegetables without added fat and sauces.	All vegetables with added fat and sauces; oven-baked french fries; avocado.	Fried potatoes, such as french fries and hash browns; vegetables fried in oil.
Fruits	Fresh and frozen fruits; fruits canned in their juice.	100% fruit juice; fruits canned in light syrup; dried fruits.	Fruits canned in heavy syrup.
Breads and Cereals	Whole-grain bread, pita bread; tortillas; pasta; brown rice; whole-grain cereals with no added sugar.	White refined-flour bread, rice, and pasta; french toast; taco shells; corn bread; biscuits; waffles; pancakes; granola.	Croissants; muffins; doughnuts; sweet rolls; cereals with added sugar.
Milk and Milk Products	Fat-free or 1% milk; fat-free or low-fat yogurt; part-skim, reduced-fat, and fat-free cheese; low-fat or fat-free cottage cheese.	2% low-fat milk; processed cheese spread.	Whole milk; cheese (such as American, cheddar, and Swiss); cream cheese; yogurt made with whole milk.

Category			
Meats, Chicken, Fish, Eggs, Beans, and Nuts	Trimmed beef and pork; extra lean ground beef; chicken and turkey without skin; tuna canned in water; baked, broiled, steamed, and grilled fish; beans; split peas; lentils.	Lean ground beef, broiled hamburgers; ham; chicken and turkey with skin; tuna canned in oil; peanut butter; nuts.	Untrimmed beef and pork; regular ground beef; fried hamburgers; ribs; bacon; fried chicken, chicken nuggets; hot dogs; lunch meats; pepperoni; sausage; fried fish.
Sweets and Snacks	Frozen fruit juice bars; low-fat frozen yogurt and ice-cream; fig bars; baked chips; low-fat popcorn; pretzels.		Cookies; cakes; pies; ice cream; chocolate; candy; chips; buttered popcorn.
Fats (stuff that goes on or in your food)	Ketchup; mustard; fat-free salad dressing; fat-free mayonnaise; fat-free sour cream; vegetable oil; olive oil; oil-based salad dressing.	Low-fat salad dressing; low-fat mayonnaise; low-fat sour cream.	Butter; margarine; gravy; regular creamy salad dressing; mayonnaise; tartar sauce; sour cream; cream sauce; cheese sauce; cream sauce.
Drinks	Water; diet soda; diet lemonade.	100% fruit juice; sports drinks.	Regular soda; sweetened iced tea; lemonade; fruit drinks with less than 100% fruit juice.

2 to 3 servings per day from the *meats, chicken, fish, eggs, beans, and nuts* food group and 2 to 3 servings per day from the *milk and milk products* food group will supply all the protein your body needs.

Your ability to tone your body and build muscular strength depends on your age, how regularly you exercise, and whether you eat nutritious food. Extra servings of protein-rich foods or protein supplements won't help because your body doesn't store extra protein. Your body converts the excess protein and stores it as body fat.

Obesity

Being a few pounds overweight doesn't mean you're obese. It is a good indication, though, that you are eating more calories than your body is using. There are many possible reasons for this, including poor eating habits, overeating, not getting enough exercise, family history, illness, stress, low self-esteem, and emotional problems.

Being too overweight, however, is a serious problem for some young men. As a result, they can suffer from high blood pressure, diabetes, heart disease, bone and joint problems, breathing problems, sleeping problems, and liver and gall bladder disease.

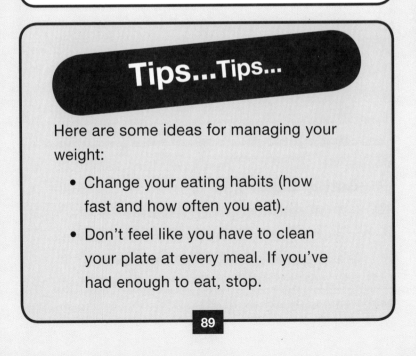

Tips...Tips...

Here are some ideas for managing your weight:

- Change your eating habits (how fast and how often you eat).
- Don't feel like you have to clean your plate at every meal. If you've had enough to eat, stop.

- Eat less fatty food, and avoid junk and fast foods.
- Control your portion size and consume fewer calories.
- Increase your physical activity.
- Don't eat meals in front of the TV or computer.
- Don't reward yourself with food for a job well-done.
- Limit snacks.
- Work with your doctor to monitor your weight and start a weight-management program if necessary.

Eating Disorders

Sometimes, young men can be underweight because of a health problem, like anorexia or bulimia. Often there is a link between eating disorders and the desire for athletic ability. If you want physical perfection too much, it can cause life-threatening behaviors connected to your diet, use of food supplements, and approach to exercise.

Be aware of your behavior if you participate in sports that require you to be thin to excel. If you're a runner, for example, you're more likely to have an eating disorder than if you're a football player. Wrestlers who try to quickly shed pounds before a match so they can compete in a lower weight category are at especially high risk, too. Just be careful out there!

Anabolic Steroids

Anabolic steroids are man-made drugs available legally only by prescription. Using anabolic steroids leads to serious, irreversible health problems. Some people, especially some athletes, abuse anabolic steroids to enhance their performance and improve their physical appearance. And users often combine several different types of steroids to maximize their effectiveness.

But it's important to know that there are a number of serious and dangerous side effects from using anabolic steroids. Here are a few:

- Liver tumors and cancer.
- Kidney tumors.
- Jaundice (yellowish pigmentation of skin, tissues, and body fluid).
- High blood pressure.
- Severe acne.
- Nervous trembling.
- Shrinking of the testicles.
- Baldness.
- Development of breasts.
- Prostate cancer.

- Increases in LDL (bad cholesterol).
- Decreases in HDL (good cholesterol).
- Added risk of contracting HIV/AIDS or hepatitis through needle use.

There are even more dangers for young men like you. Using anabolic steroids can stop you from growing to your full height. This means that you will risk remaining shorter than you would have been had you not taken them.

Some food supplements contain anabolic steroids. You can see advertisements for them on the Internet or in bodybuilding magazines. Some of the supplements are legal and others are illegal. But legal or illegal, these supplements can cause health problems.

Heard enough? Well, here's the bottom line: Don't use anabolic steroids!

BODY CARE

Good Personal Hygiene Looks Good

Lots of people think young men are laid-back when it comes to their appearance. But it's a fact that guys spend a lot of time in front of the mirror. What's wrong with looking your best?

A young man who appreciates the value of being fit also takes pride in his physique and general appearance. Little things like brushing your teeth after breakfast and shampooing your hair regularly influence how you see yourself and how others see you.

There are no halfway measures when it comes to personal hygiene. A young man may be freshly bathed and neatly dressed, but his look is spoiled if he neglects to comb his hair or his fingernails are dirty. You'll get the most out of the time and effort you spend to be physically fit if you establish basic personal hygiene habits now.

Body Hygiene

Keep your body clean with a gentle soap. It's a good idea to shower or bathe every day, especially after exercising. Clean under your arms, between your toes, behind your ears, and all around your groin. Wash your face, too. As you enter puberty and your skin gets oilier, it's a good idea to wash your face two or three times a day with soap and warm water. There are lots of skin-care cleansers, but unless you have a special problem (like really dry skin or bad acne), a gentle soap is really all you need to do the job.

There are special sweat glands that start working for the first time when you start puberty. These glands are found only under your arms and around your genitals. The sweat from them contains proteins and carbohydrates that mix with the bacteria on your skin to cause a bad smell. Showering with warm water and cleaning with a mild soap will wash away the bacteria and help control your body odor.

It's also a good time to start using a deodorant or antiperspirant. The difference between deodorants and antiperspirants is that deodorants cover up the smell while antiperspirants stop or dry up the sweat. They are two different ways to solve the same problem. Try both and see which you like best.

Take care of your hair. It's not so important whether it's long or short or somewhere in-between. What matters is that your hair is clean and well groomed. That means shampooing it regularly to keep it from getting oily and greasy to the touch. It also means regular trips to the barber to keep it looking neat.

Before you know it, the hair on your face will start to grow. Most young men begin to shave every few days once puberty begins. As time goes by, your facial hair will get thicker and grow more quickly. One day you may decide to try growing a beard or mustache. Until then, though, look sharp by shaving to keep your face smooth and clean looking.

And don't forget your feet. Wash them daily to keep away the fungus that causes athlete's foot. After showering and bathing, dry your feet really well—especially between your toes. And don't wear the same pair of shoes and socks day after day. If you do get athlete's foot, it's easy to treat with any of the sprays, powders, or creams available at the drugstore. Also keep your toenails trimmed, cutting straight across to avoid ingrown nails, which are painful and can get infected.

Oral Hygiene

Your mouth—and everything in it—is a very important part of your personal hygiene. Good oral hygiene is when your mouth looks and smells healthy. This means your gums are pink, your teeth are clean and free of food, and you don't have bad breath. Good oral health makes you look and feel good, and helps you eat and speak properly.

Only flossing can clean between your teeth and under your gums. A toothbrush can't do it. Flossing also scrapes plaque from the surface of your teeth and from under your gums. Plaque is a film of germs that live in your mouth and stick to your teeth. Plaque causes tooth decay and gum disease.

Brush your teeth any way that works for you. Just don't scrub hard back and forth; doing that can damage your gums and tooth enamel. Most people find that small circular motions and short back and forth motions work best. And don't forget to brush your tongue. It collects bacteria and dead cells that cause gum disease and bad breath.

Choose the right toothbrush. The best ones have soft, nylon, round-ended bristles. Hard bristles can injure your gums and the enamel on your teeth. And be sure that your brush is the right size for your mouth. Small-headed brushes are better since they can reach every part of your mouth, including your back teeth.

It's also important that you use the right toothpaste. Select toothpaste that contains fluoride. Fluoride protects your teeth from decay. Ask your dentist which toothpaste is right for you if you're not sure. And remember, you need only a squirt about the size of a pea to do the job right.

Sleep Hygiene

Sleep is how your body recharges itself so you'll be ready to get up tomorrow feeling rested, healthy, and strong. Most young men between the ages of 8 and 12 need about 10 hours of sleep every night. The older you get, the less sleep you need. If you're between the ages of 13 and 17 you'll need about 9 hours of sleep. And if you're 18 or older, 8 hours should do it.

The best sleep is uninterrupted by disturbances like noises and pets, and it begins and ends at the same time each day. When you sleep through the night and wake up refreshed, it's what is called good sleep hygiene. Between early school start times, after-school activities, homework, and everything else going on, it can be hard to find time to get the sleep your body needs. Try hard, though; it's important that you get enough rest so you can be your best at school, in sports, and in life.

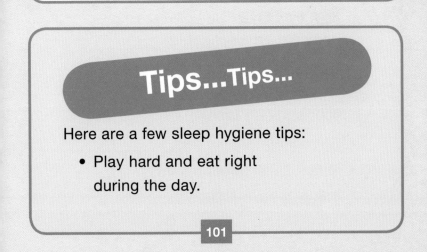

Tips...Tips...

Here are a few sleep hygiene tips:

- Play hard and eat right during the day.

- After dinner, limit foods and drinks that contain caffeine, like chocolate and sodas.

- Don't watch scary TV shows or play action video games close to bedtime because they can make it hard to sleep.

- Tune out all noise when it's time to fall asleep. Turn off your MP3 player, computer, and TV.

- Turn off the lights, like your desk lamp or a flickering computer monitor.

- Go to bed around the same time every night; this helps your body get on a schedule.

- Floss, brush, and take a warm shower every night; this tells your body it's time for bed.

- Get comfortable in bed.

- Relax. Think about things that make you happy.

PUTTING IT ALL TOGETHER

Making It Work

When you first meet someone, it's natural that they judge you by your appearance. How you dress and present yourself affects how people view and treat you. How much your clothes cost is not important. What counts is that you are clean, neat, and well groomed. The following story says it all:

> *The owner of a sales company made some observations about young men applying for their first job. "First," he said, "I watch the*

way the young man carries himself as he walks into my office for the interview. I can spot someone who is physically fit every time. When he sits down, I look at his haircut and his fingernails. Then I walk around him and glance at the back of this shirt collar to see if it's clean. As I sit down again, I offer him a cigarette to find out whether he smokes. The last thing I do is study his facial expressions and eyes. It isn't his features that interest me, as he was born with them. What I'm interested in is his composure, demeanor, and self-confidence. I don't care whether his clothes cost $20 or $200, as long as he is neatly dressed. I do all these things to find out if he is physically fit and practices good personal hygiene. If I'm satisfied that he does, then I explore his mind."

So There You Have It

This book is about your physical fitness and health. We've covered all the basics, including exercise, eating right, and caring for your body. By making your quest for fitness and health a way of life, you will have confidence and self-esteem. And in the years ahead, you will reap the benefits of forming healthy habits now. Good luck!

7-DAY EXERCISE PROGRAM

Begin with this 7-day exercise program. It's a good basic routine with just the right balance of stretching, aerobic, and resistance exercises. The program is an easy way to start because no special equipment or weights are needed; you use only your body weight for resistance.

You'll soon begin to see your flexibility, endurance, and strength develop as you follow the day-by-day instructions. Following the program for a few weeks will get you into the habit of regular exercise. Together with eating right and taking care of your body, this is a good first step toward being physically fit.

When the program no longer challenges you, try new aerobic and resistance exercises you read about earlier in the book and haven't yet tried. You can use dumbbells to make the resistance exercises more challenging. But, be sure to keep the weights light at first and follow the guidance on how many sets and reps to do, and when to increase the weight. Use the planning chart at the end of this chapter to design your next exercise program.

Don't forget to ask for help if you have questions. And remember it's always more fun if you exercise with a friend.

Day 1

WARM UP.
　Time: about 5 minutes.

FULL BODY STRETCH.
　Time: about 10 minutes.

AEROBIC EXERCISES.
　Time: about 30 minutes.

RESISTANCE EXERCISES.
　Time: about 20 minutes.

- Lunges. 3 sets, 8 to 12 reps each. Alternate each set with push-ups.
- Push-ups. 3 sets, 8 to 12 reps each. Alternate each set with lunges.
- Crunches. 3 sets, 8 to 12 reps each.

COOL DOWN AND STRETCH.
　Time: about 5 minutes.

Day 2

WARM UP.
   Time: about 5 minutes.

FULL BODY STRETCH.
   Time: about 10 minutes.

AEROBIC EXERCISES.
   Time: about 30 minutes

RESISTANCE EXERCISES.
   Time: 20 minutes.
- Chin-ups. 3 sets, 8 to 12 reps each.
- Side-lying leg lifts. 3 sets, 8 to 12 reps each. Alternate each set with calf raise.
- Calf raise. 3 sets, 8 to 12 reps each. Alternate each set with side-lying leg lifts.

COOL DOWN AND STRETCH.
   Time: about 5 minutes.

Day 3

STAY PHYSICALLY ACTIVE.

Day 4

WARM UP.
  Time: about 5 minutes.

FULL BODY STRETCH.
  Time: about 10 minutes.

AEROBIC EXERCISES.
  Time: about 30 minutes.

RESISTANCE EXERCISES.
  Time: about 20 minutes

- Lunges. 3 sets, 8 to 12 reps each. Alternate each set with push-ups.
- Push-ups. 3 sets, 8 to 12 reps each. Alternate each set with lunges.
- Crunches. 3 sets, 8 to 12 reps each.

COOL DOWN AND STRETCH.
  Time: about 5 minutes.

Day 5

WARM UP.
  Time: about 5 minutes.

FULL BODY STRETCH.
  Time: about 10 minutes.

AEROBIC EXERCISES.
  Time: about 30 minutes.

RESISTANCE EXERCISES.
  Time: about 30 minutes.
- Chin-ups. 3 sets, 8 to 12 reps each.
- Side-lying leg lifts. 3 sets, 8 to 12 reps each. Alternate each set with calf raise.
- Calf raise. 3 sets, 8 to 12 reps each. Alternate each set with side-lying leg lifts.

COOL DOWN AND STRETCH.
   Time: about 5 minutes.

Day 6

STAY PHYSICALLY ACTIVE.

Day 7

STAY PHYSICALLY ACTIVE.

7-DAY EXERCISE PROGRAM

Name:

Activity	Date 8/9	8/10	8/11	8/12	8/13	8/14	8/15
Warm-up	5m	5m	X	5m	5m	X	X
Full-body stretch	10m	10m	X	10m	10m	X	X
Aerobic exercises	30m	30m	X	30m	30m	X	X
Resistance exercises							
Lunges	3-8	X	X	3-8	X	X	X
Push-ups	3-8	X	X	3-8	X	X	X
Crunches	3-9	X	X	3-9	X	X	X
Chin-ups	X	3-8	X	X	3-8	X	X
Side-lying leg lifts	X	3-9	X	X	3-9	X	X
Calf raise	X	3-8	X	X	3-8	X	X
Cool down & stretch	5m	5m	X	5m	5m	X	X

Use abreviated Notes to track your daily progress. For example:

Activity	Notes

5m = 5 minutes.
3-8 = 3 sets at 8 reps each.
3|20s = 3 sets for 20 seconds each.
3-8|20 = 3 sets - 8 reps with 20 lbs.
J2|25m = Jogged 2 miles in 25 minutes.
X = Skipped / Not applicable.
↪ = Alternate.

7-DAY EXERCISE PROGRAM

Activity	Date							

Name:

7-DAY EXERCISE PROGRAM

Name:

Activity	Date							

7-DAY EXERCISE PROGRAM

Activity	Date						

Name:

7-DAY EXERCISE PROGRAM

Activity	Date						

Name:

Index